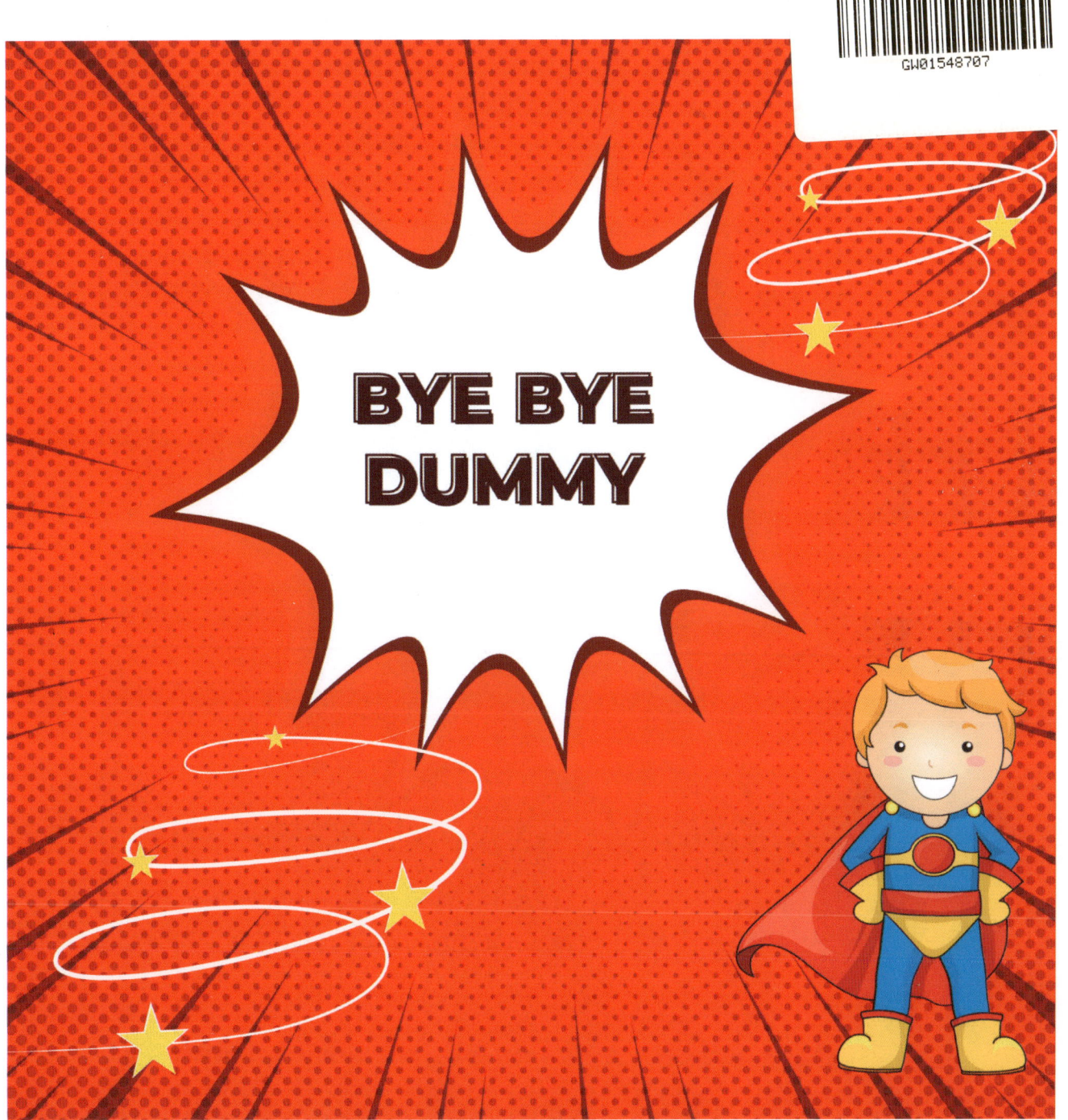

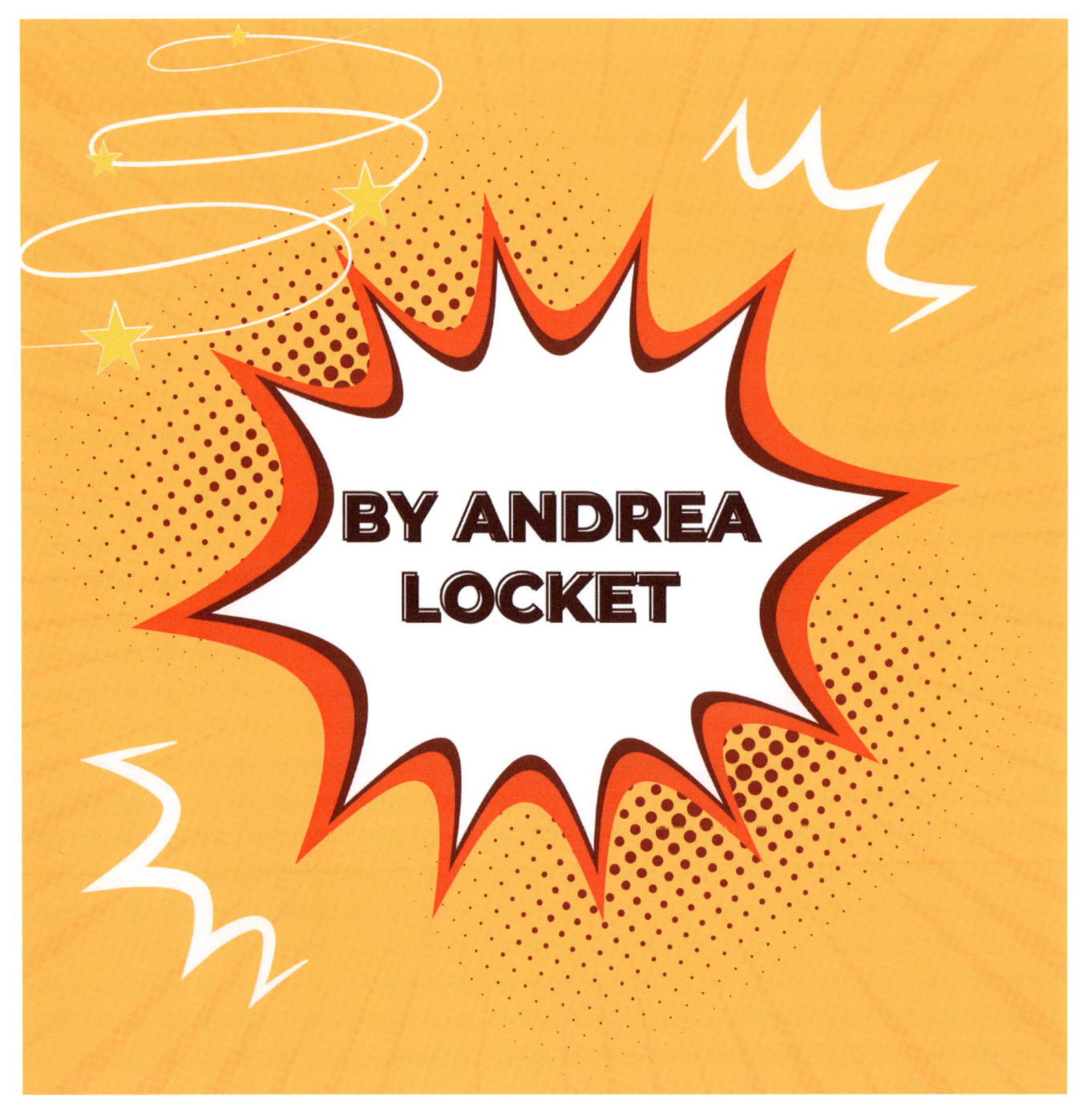

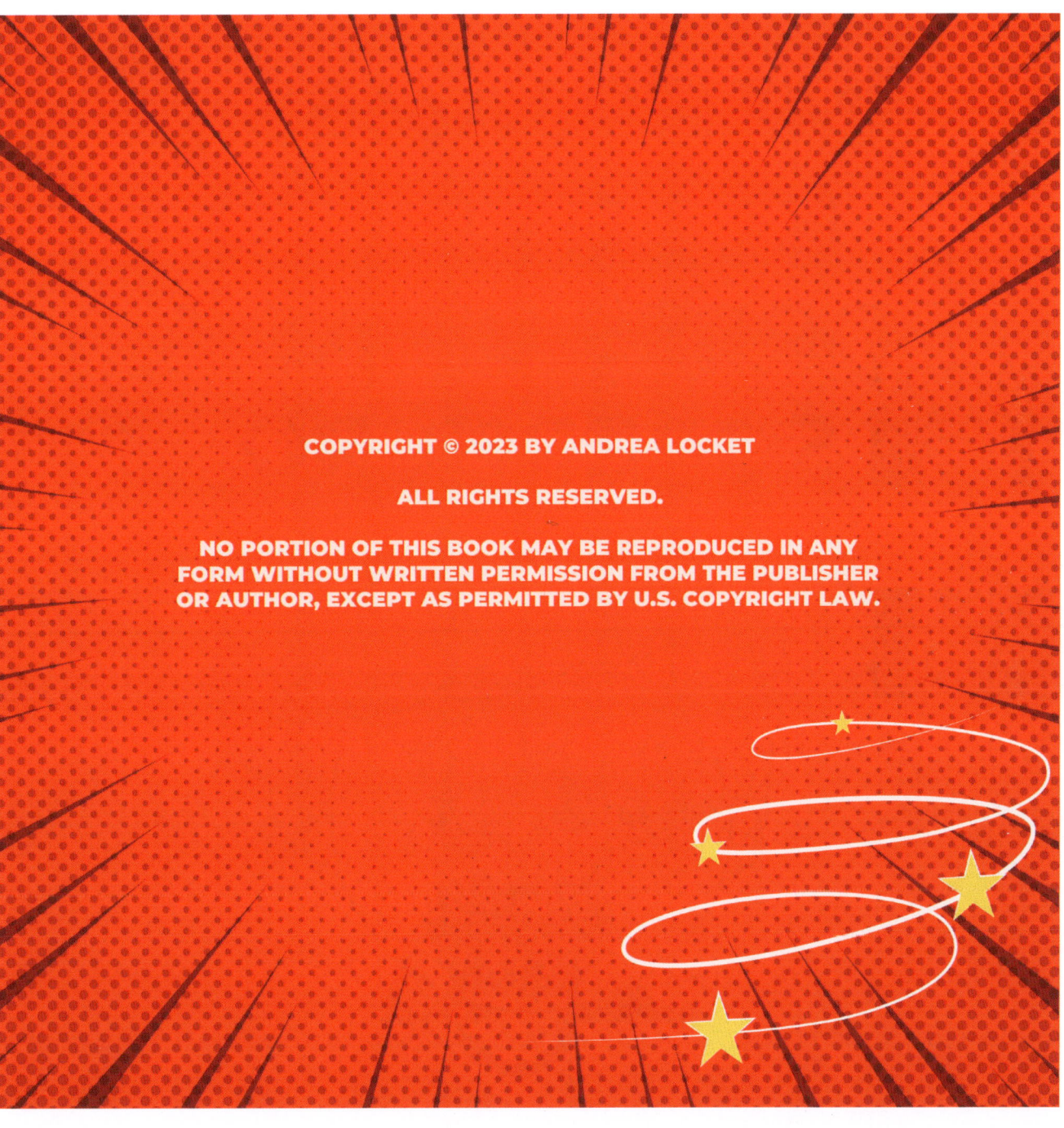

MEET JAMES - HE LOVES TO DRESS UP AS A SUPERHERO

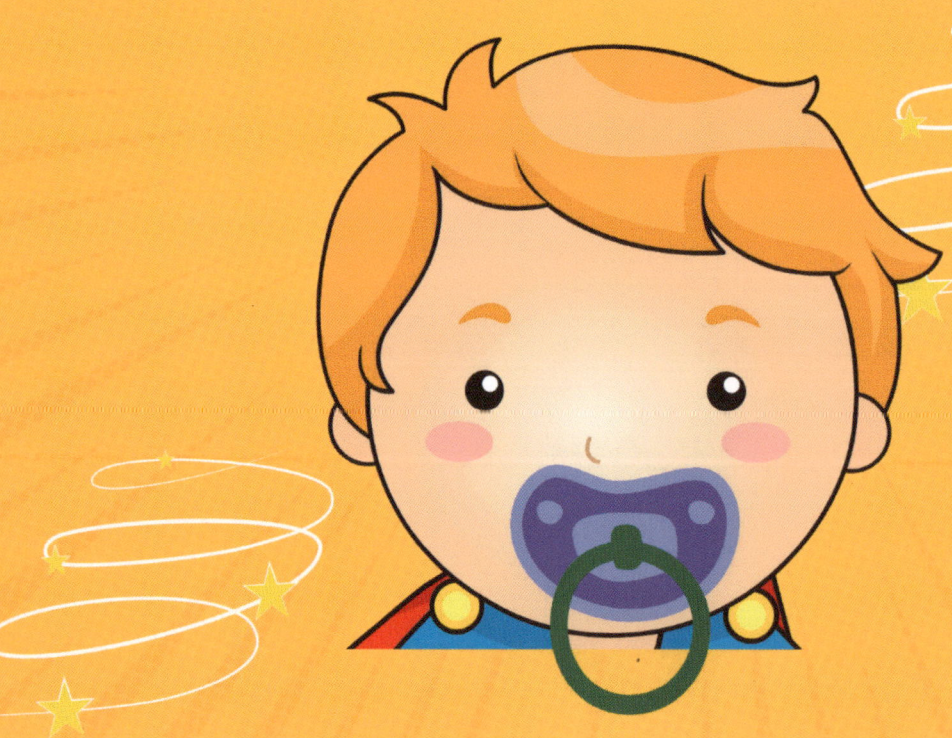

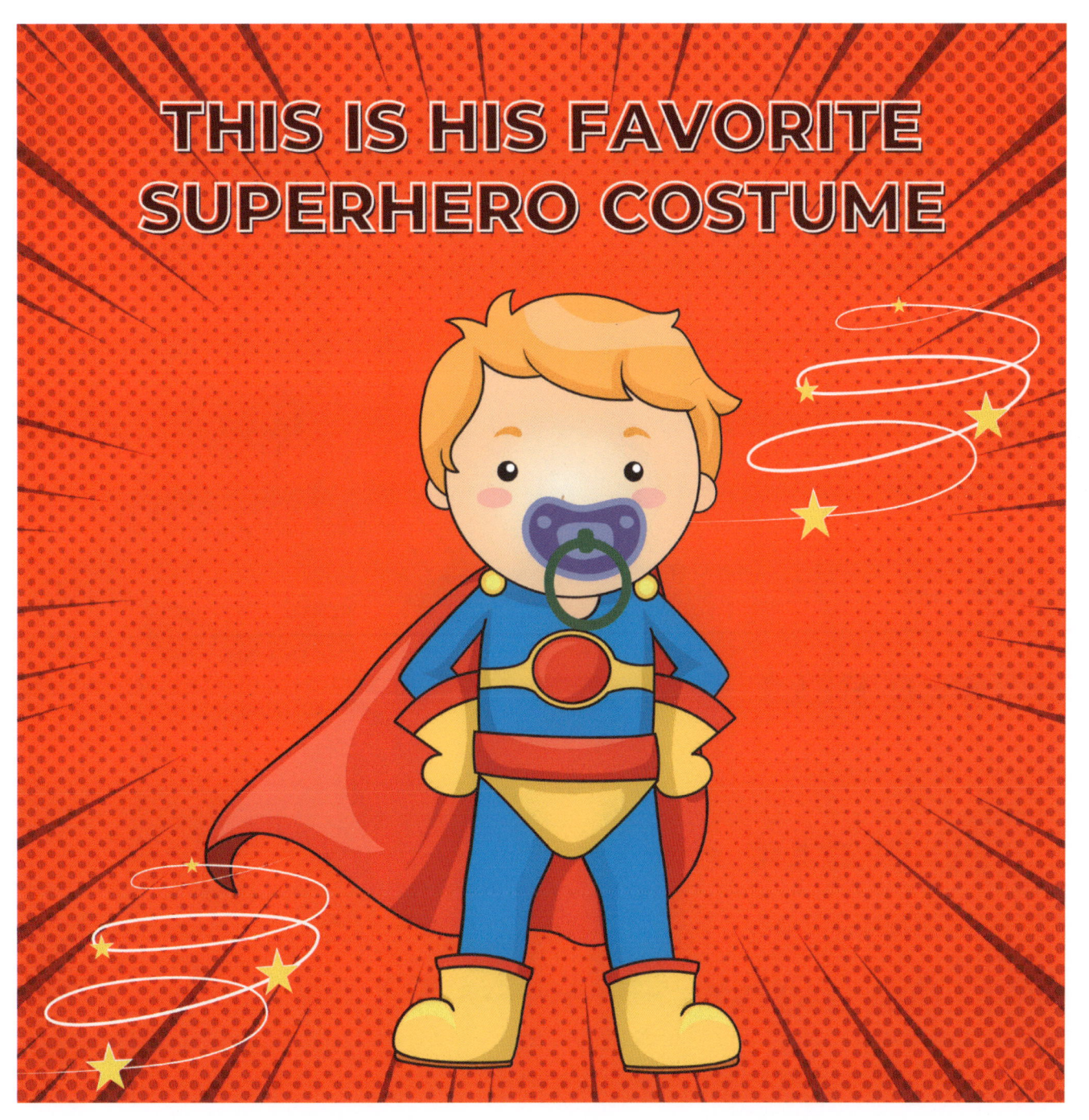

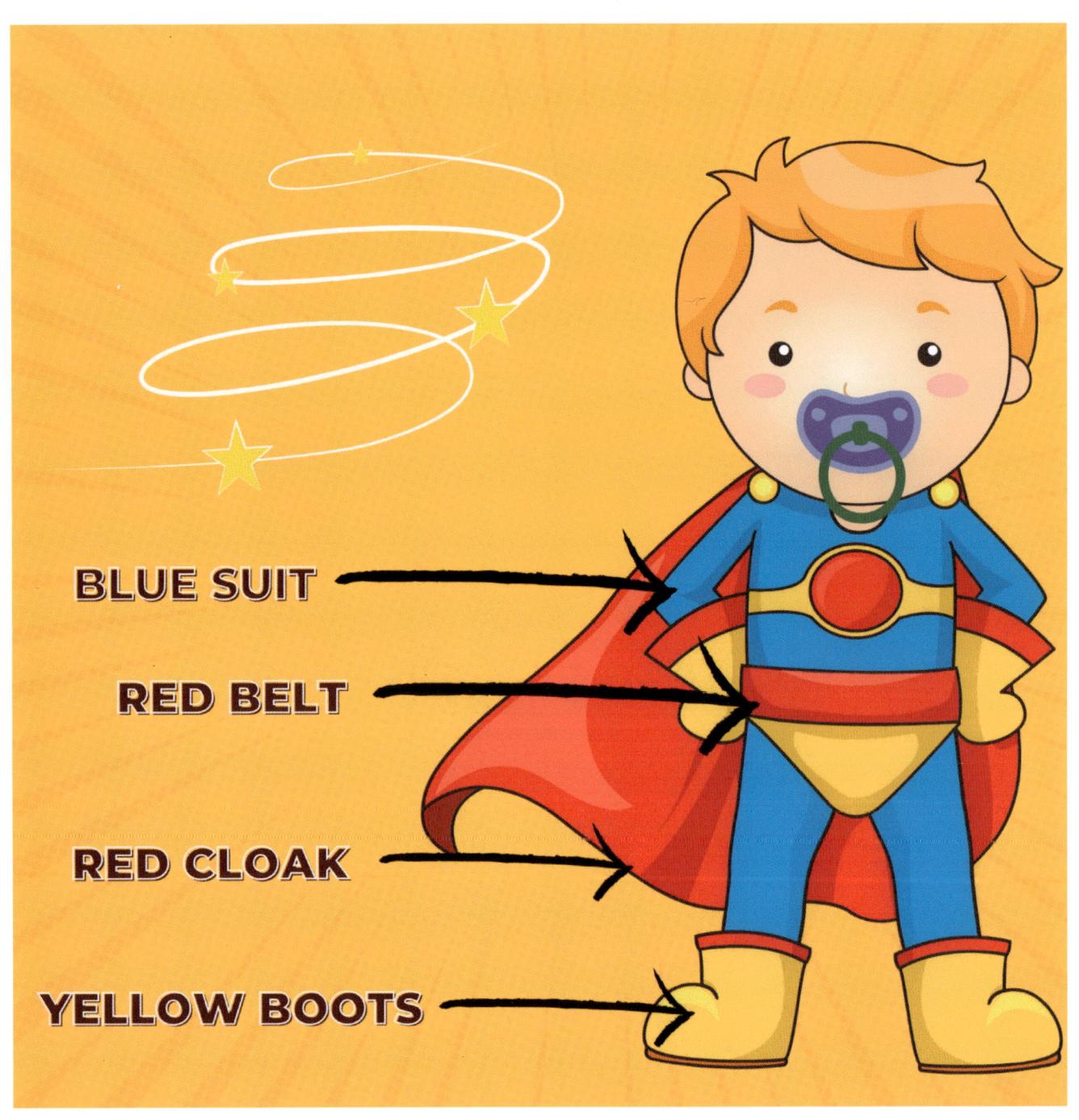

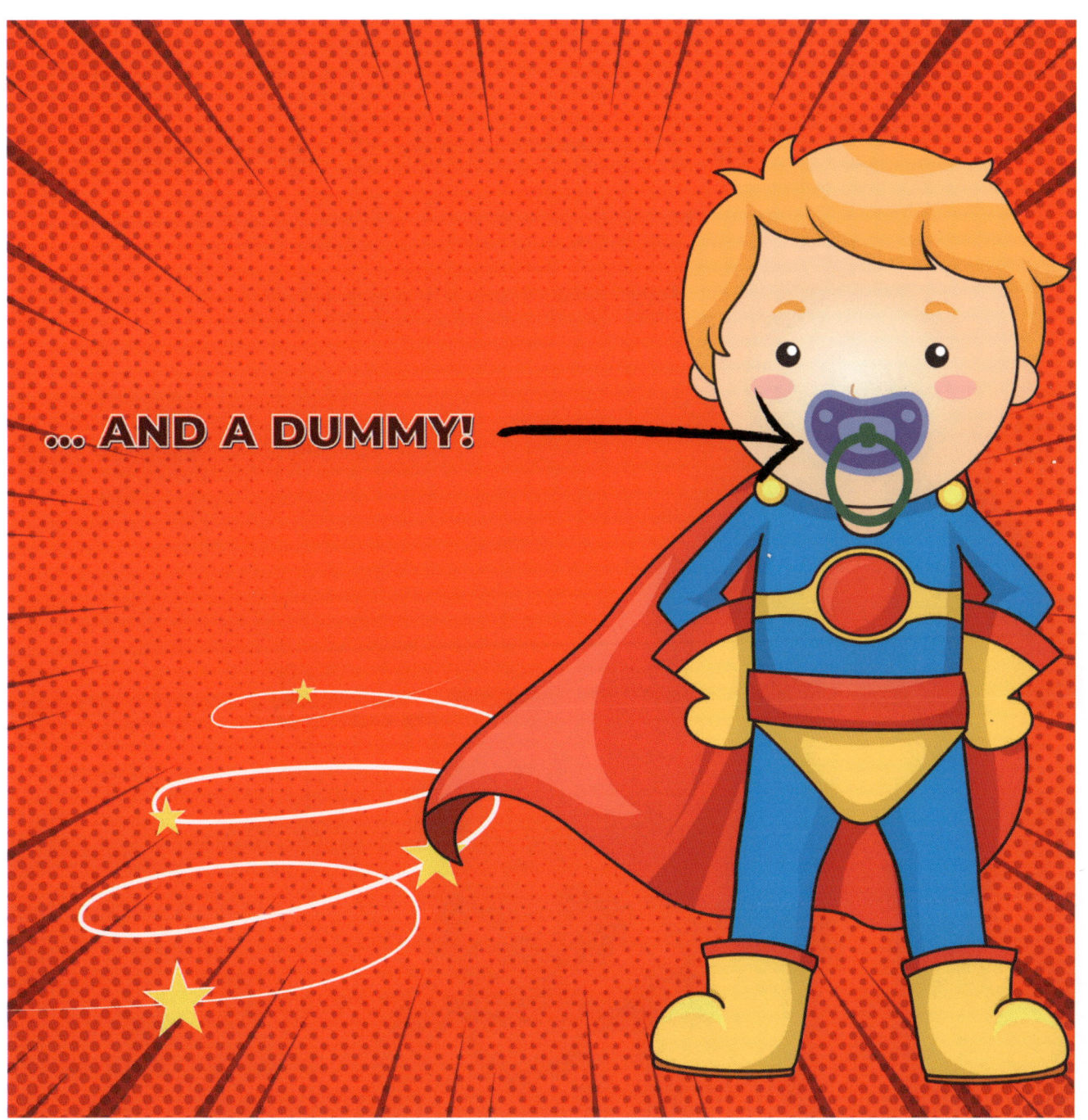

JAMES IS FAIRLY SURE SUPERHEROS DON'T HAVE DUMMIES

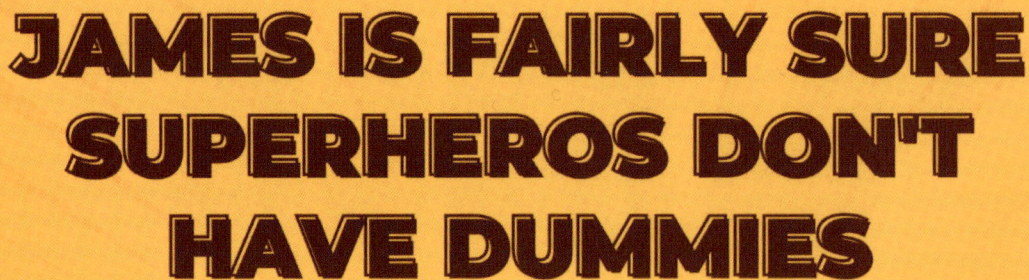

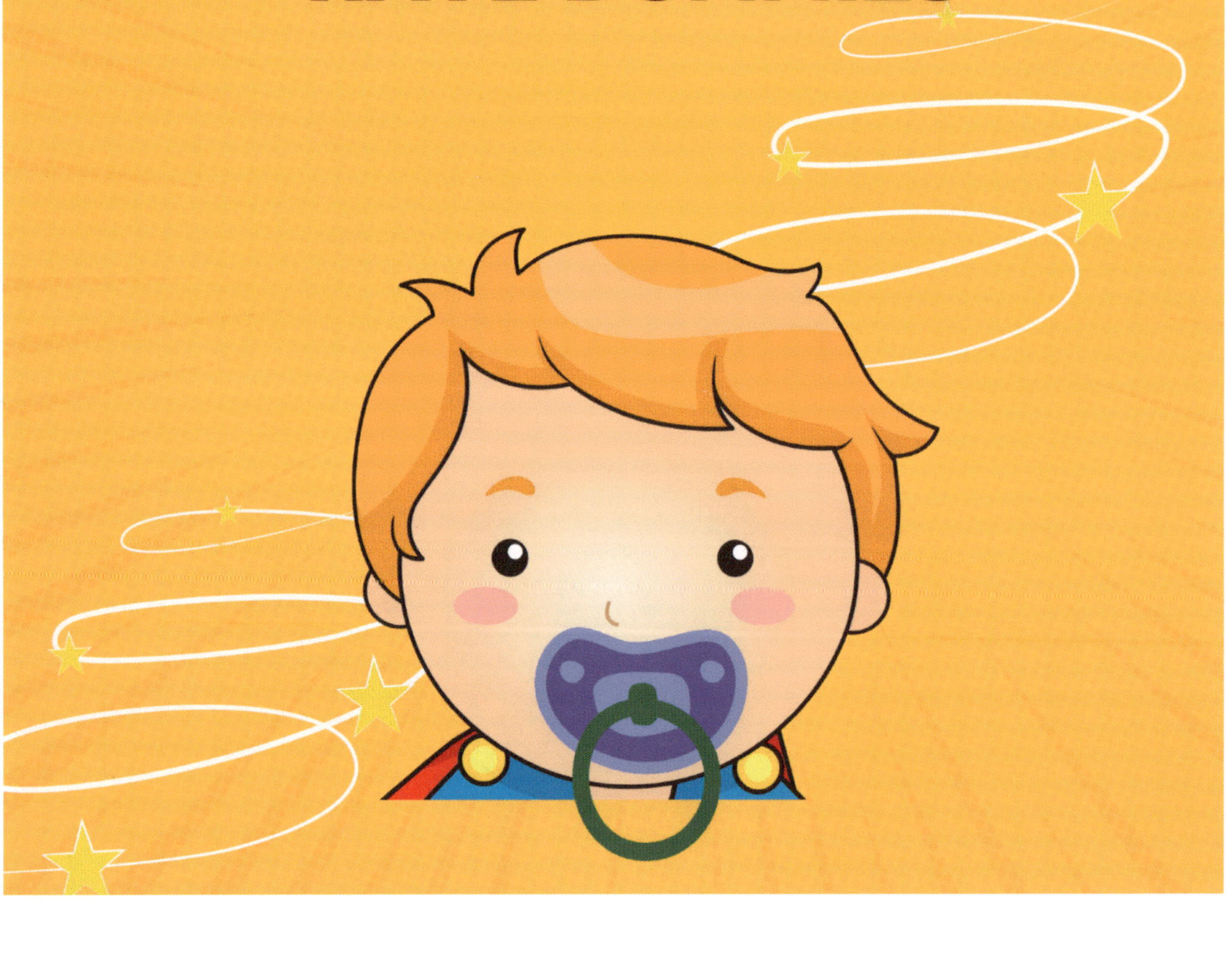

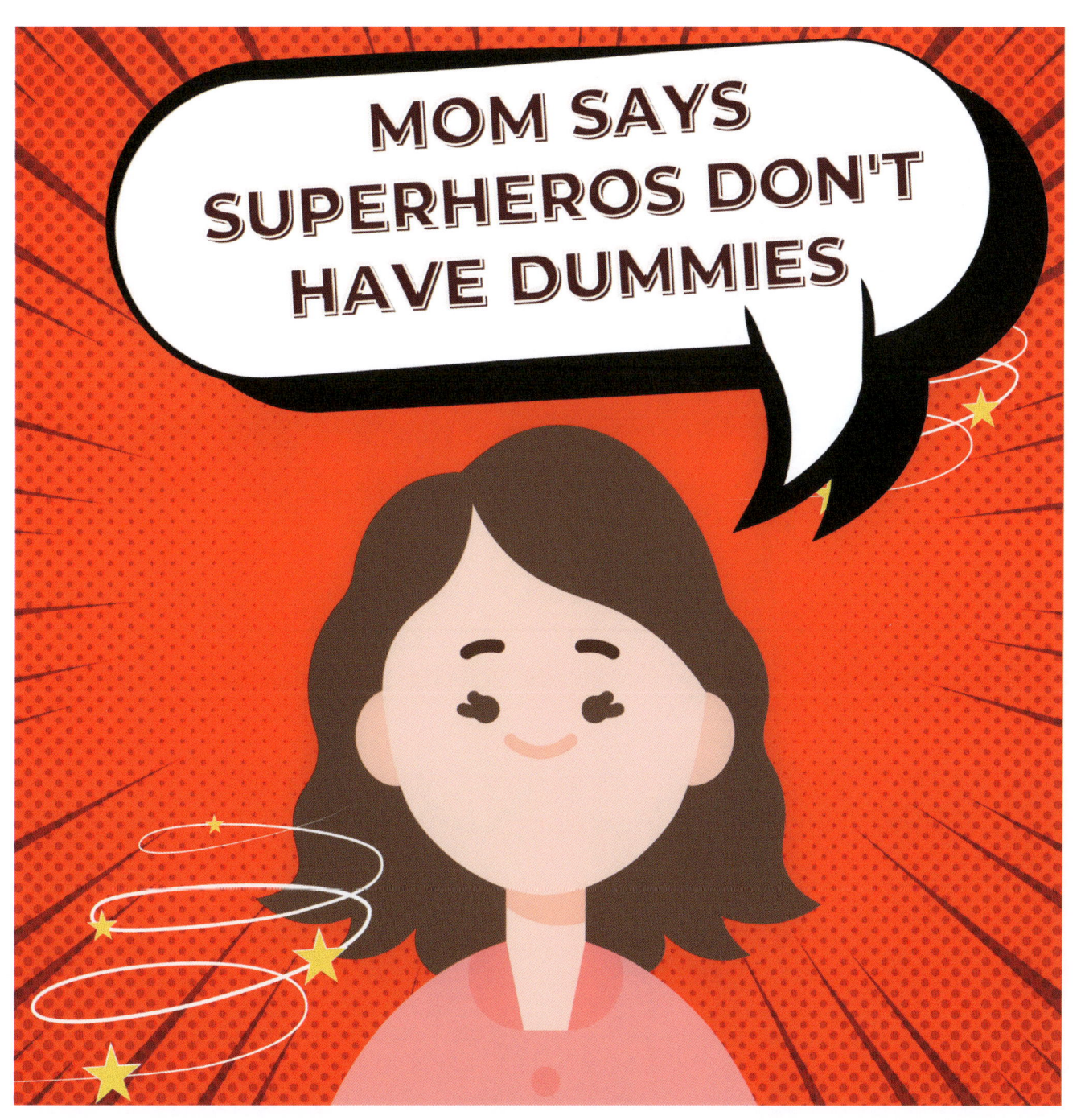

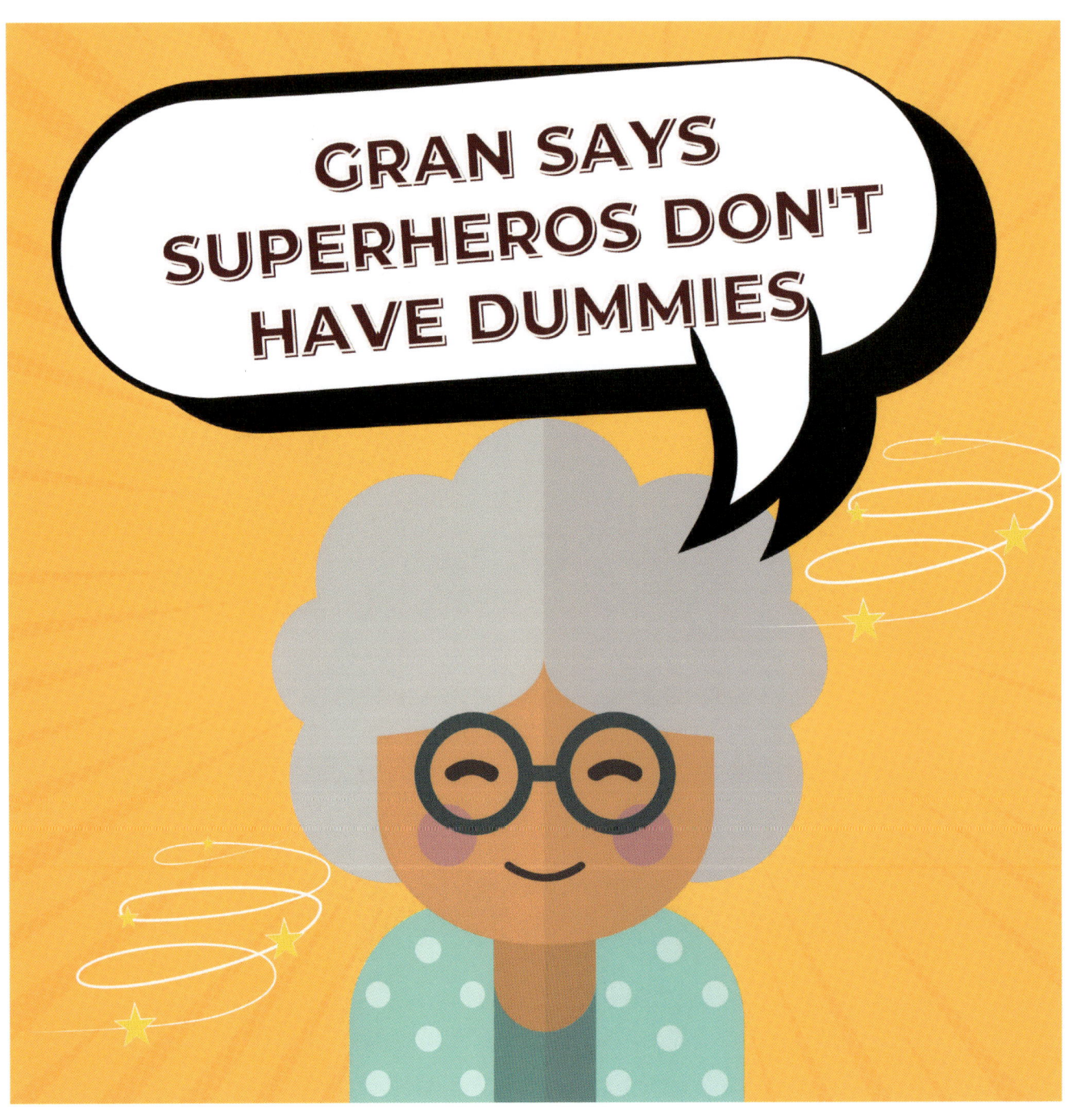

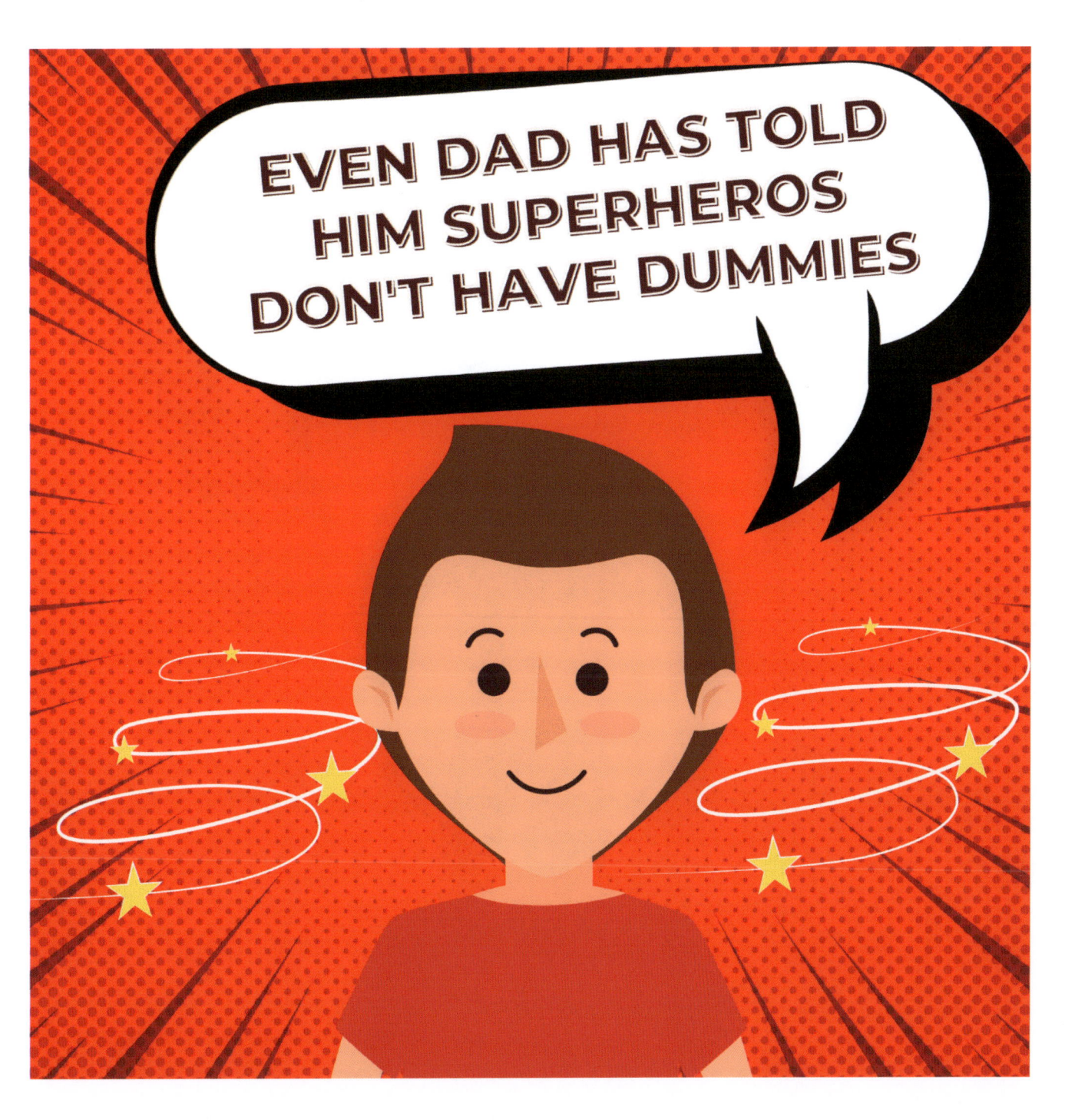

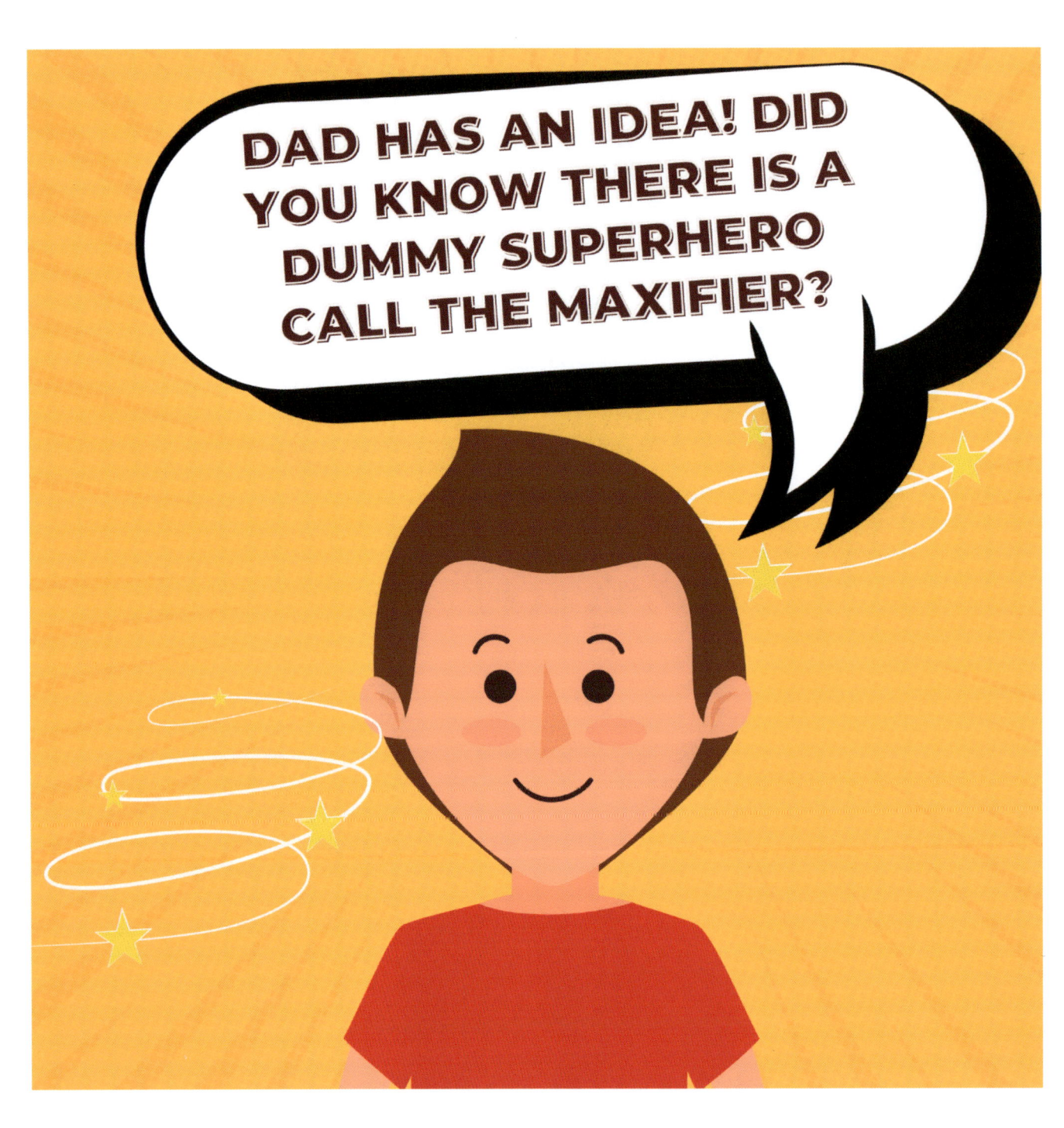

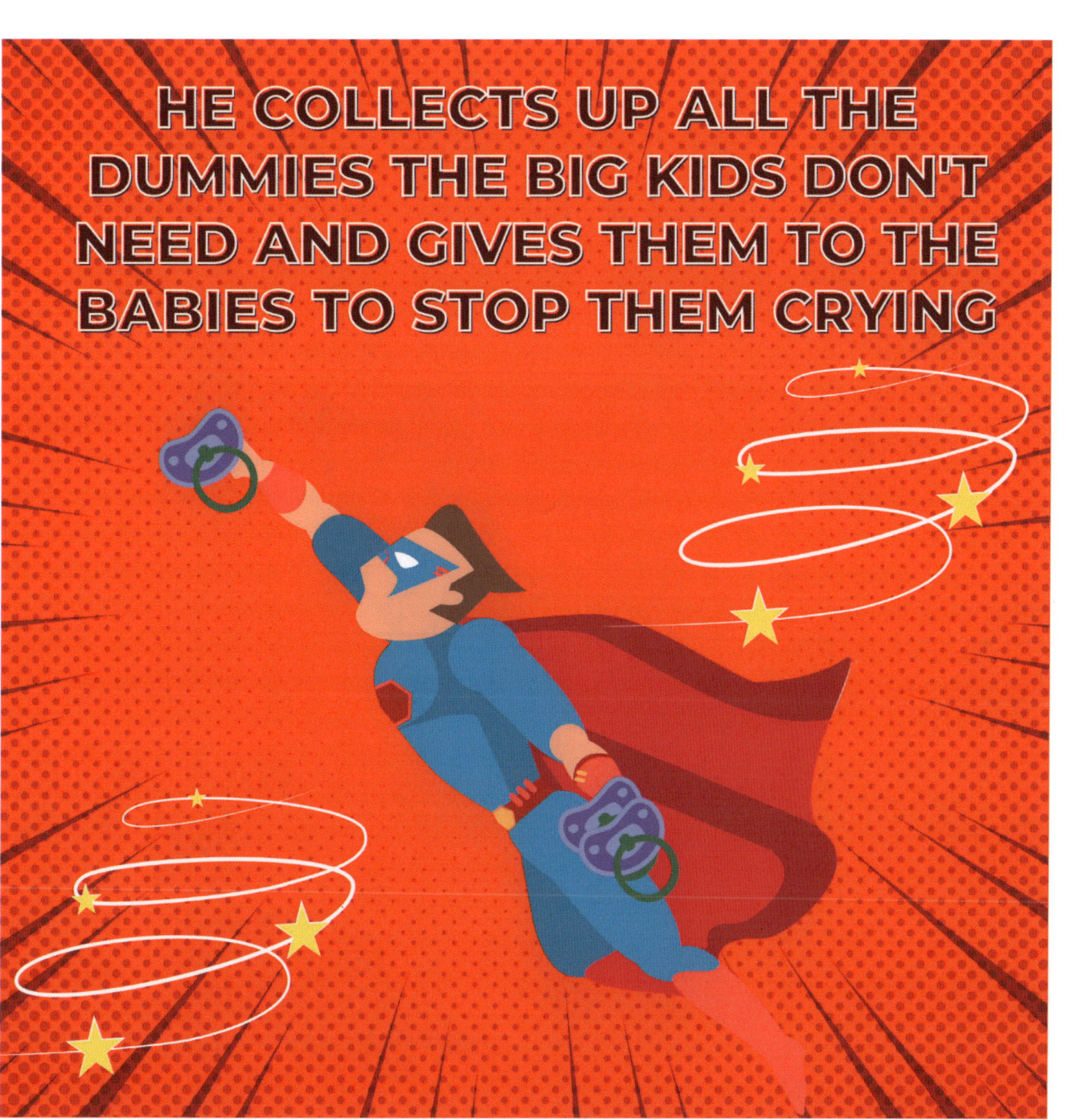

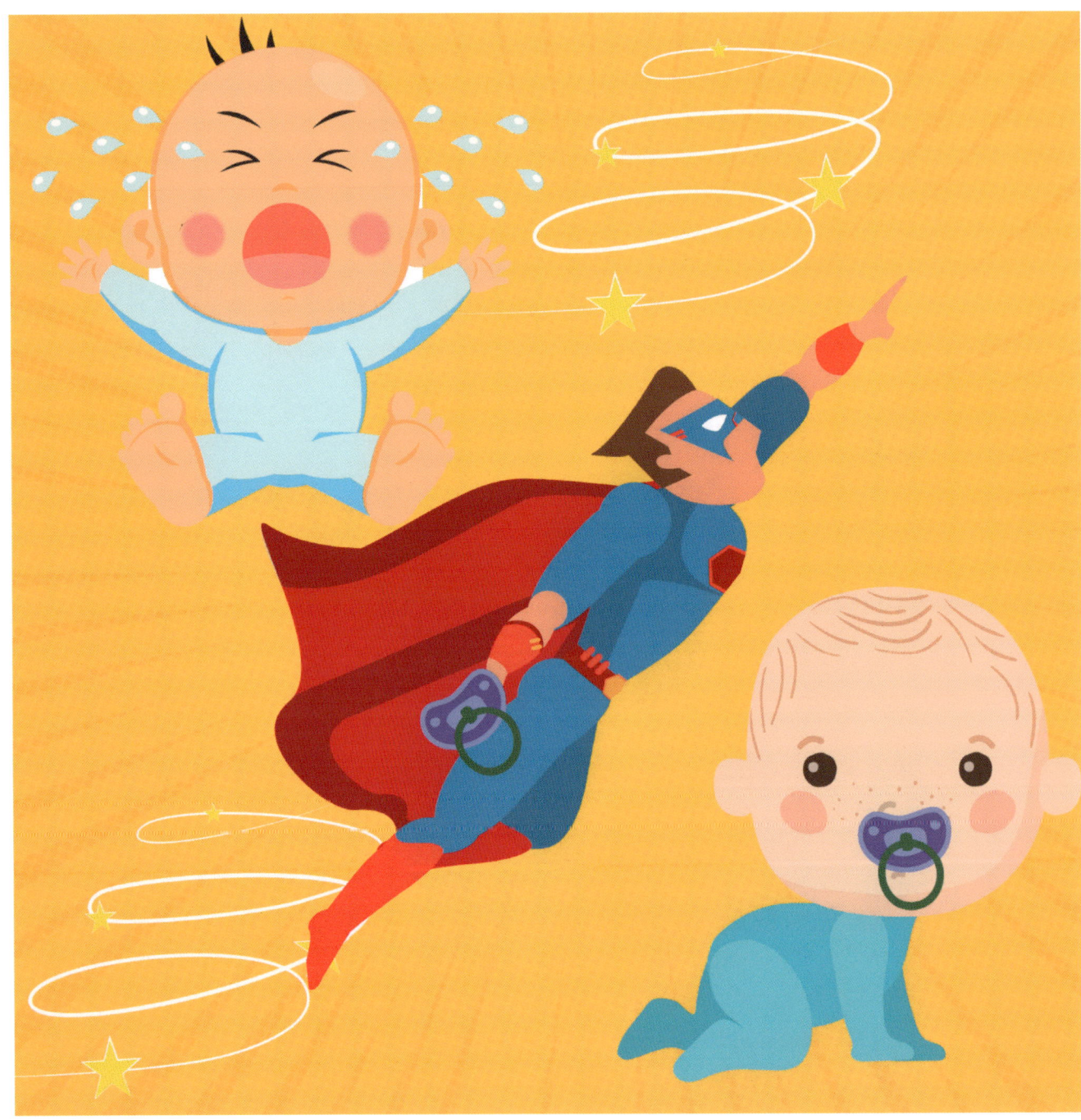

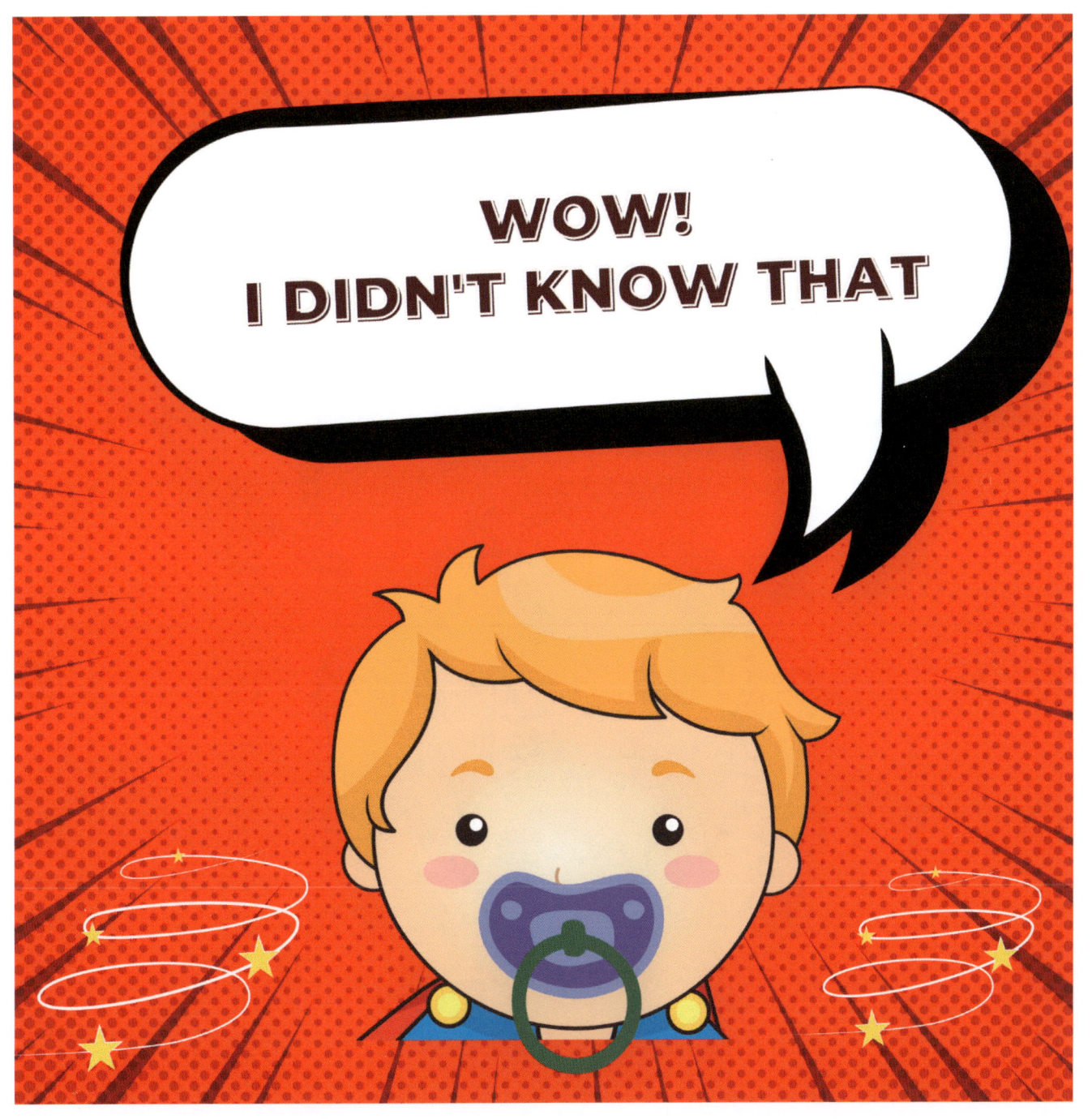

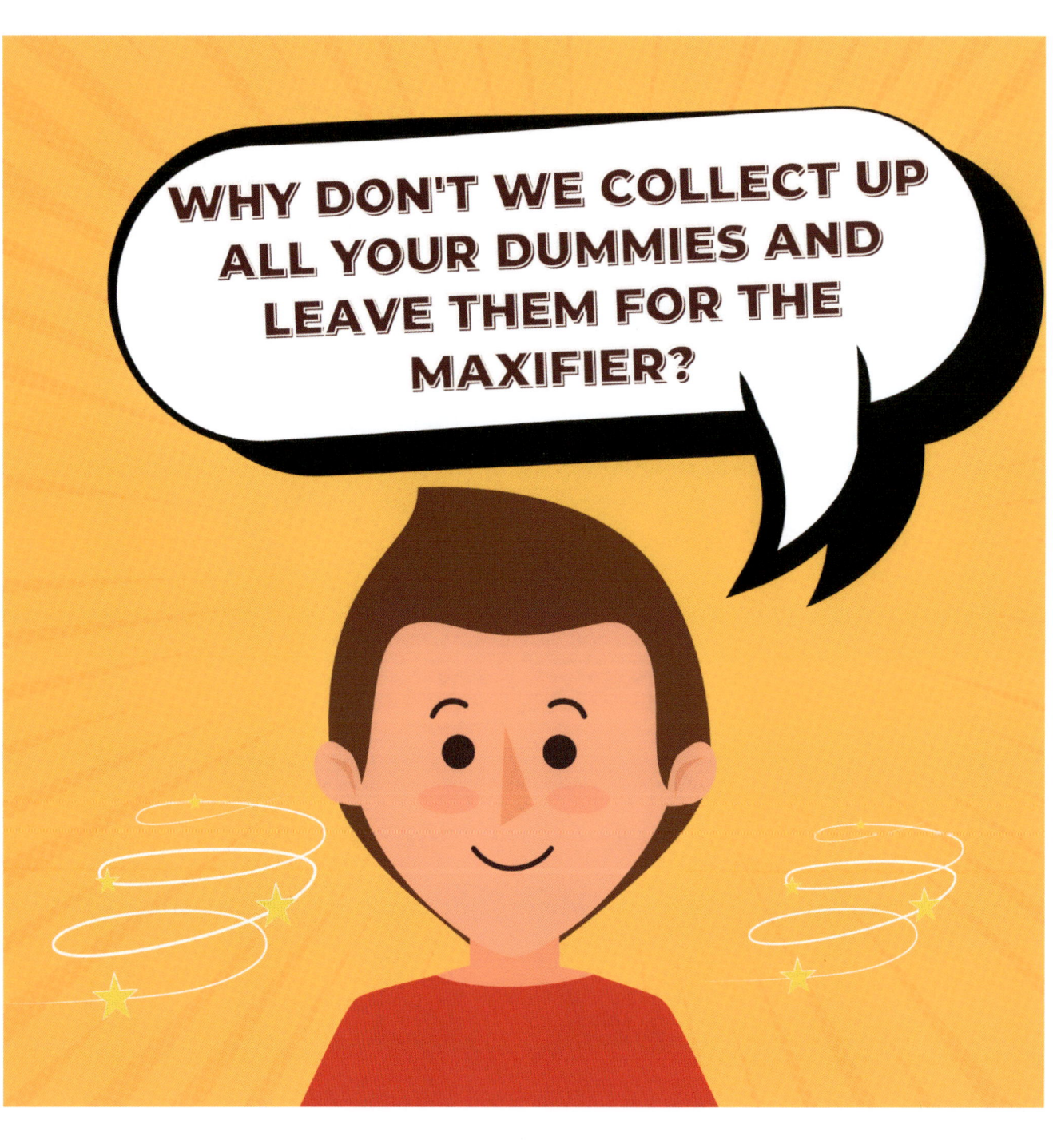

JAMES COLLECTS UP ALL HIS DUMMIES AND PUT THEM IN A BOX

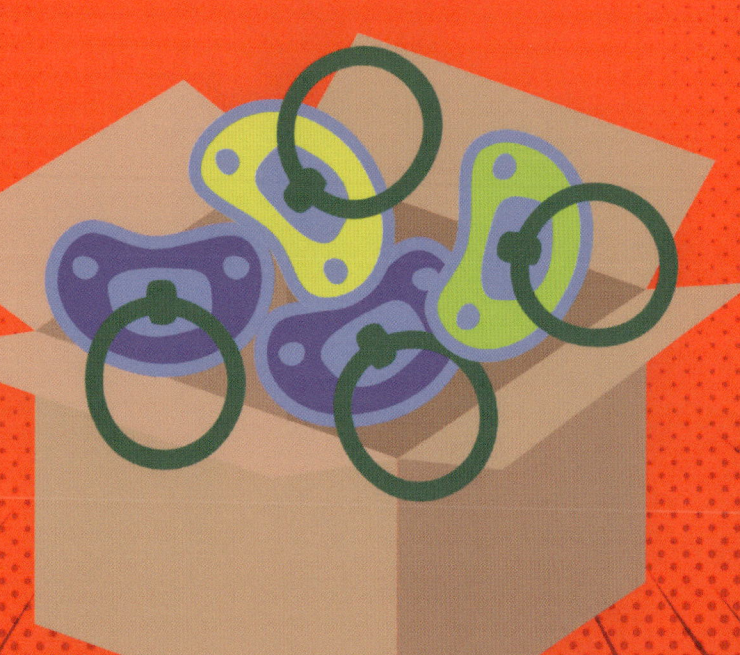

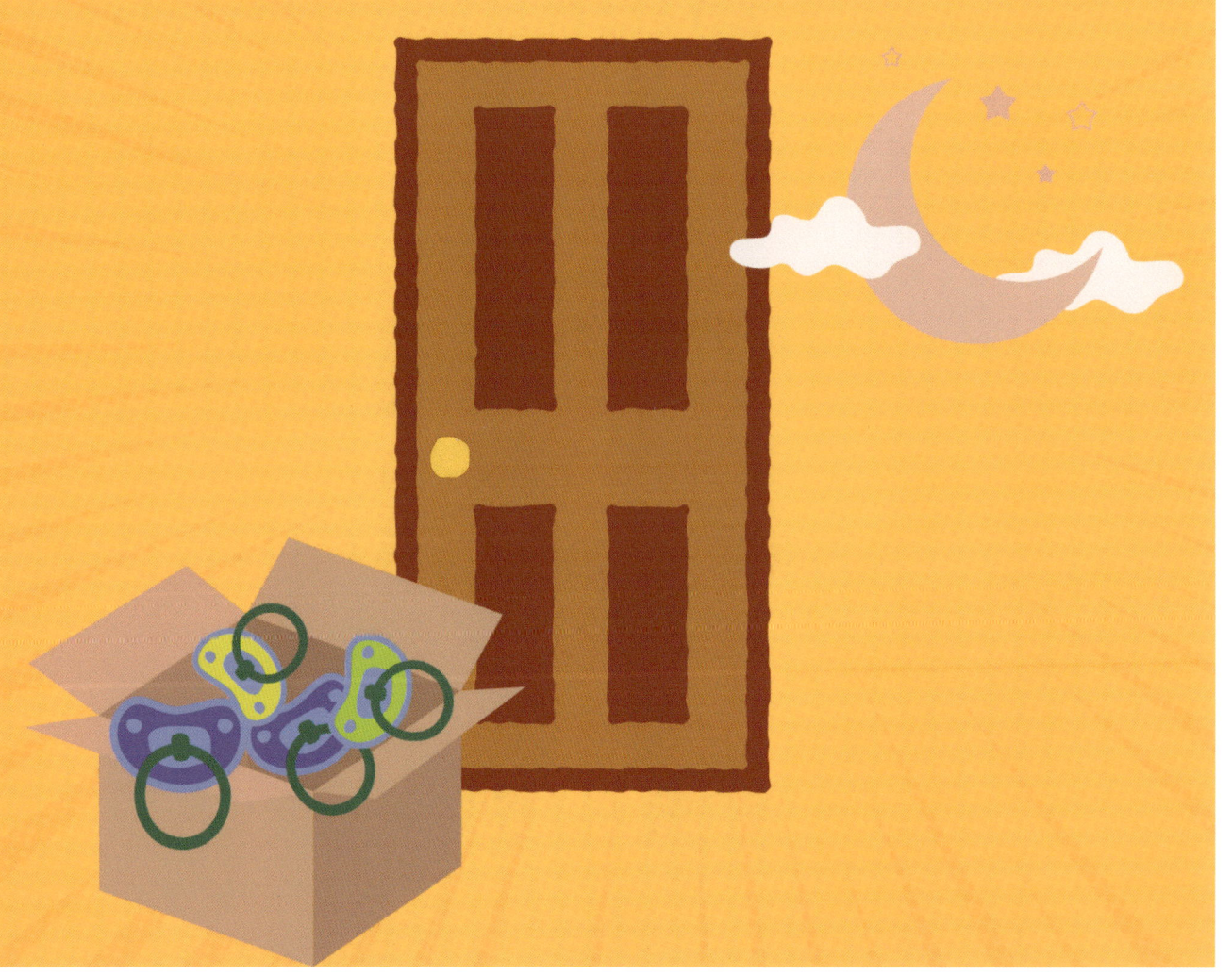

THAT NIGHT JAMES LEAVES THE BOX OUTSIDE HIS BEDROOM DOOR

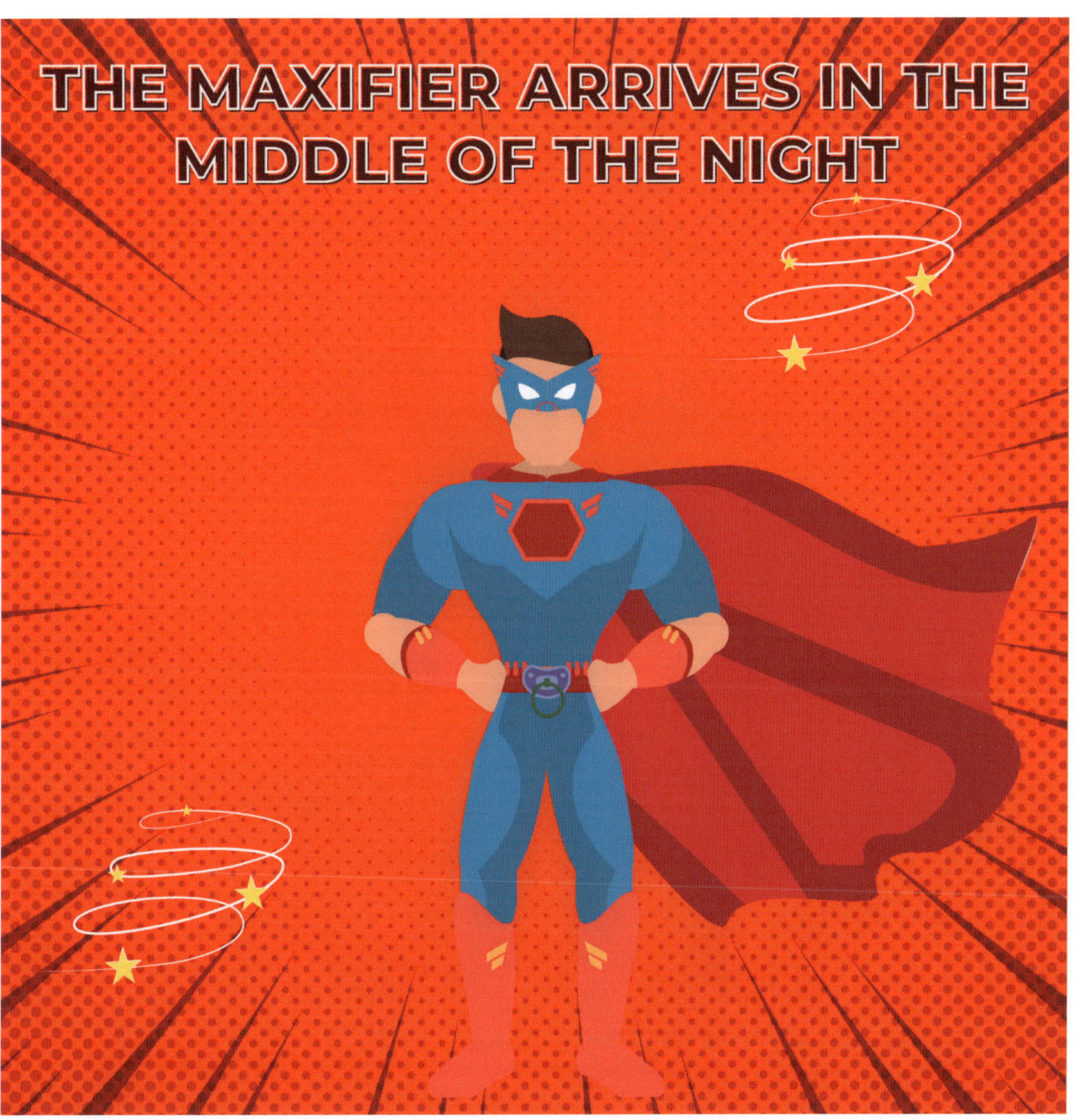

THE MAXIFIER IS SO PLEASED WITH THE BOX OF DUMMIES HE LEAVES AN EXTRA SPECIAL PRESENT FOR JAMES

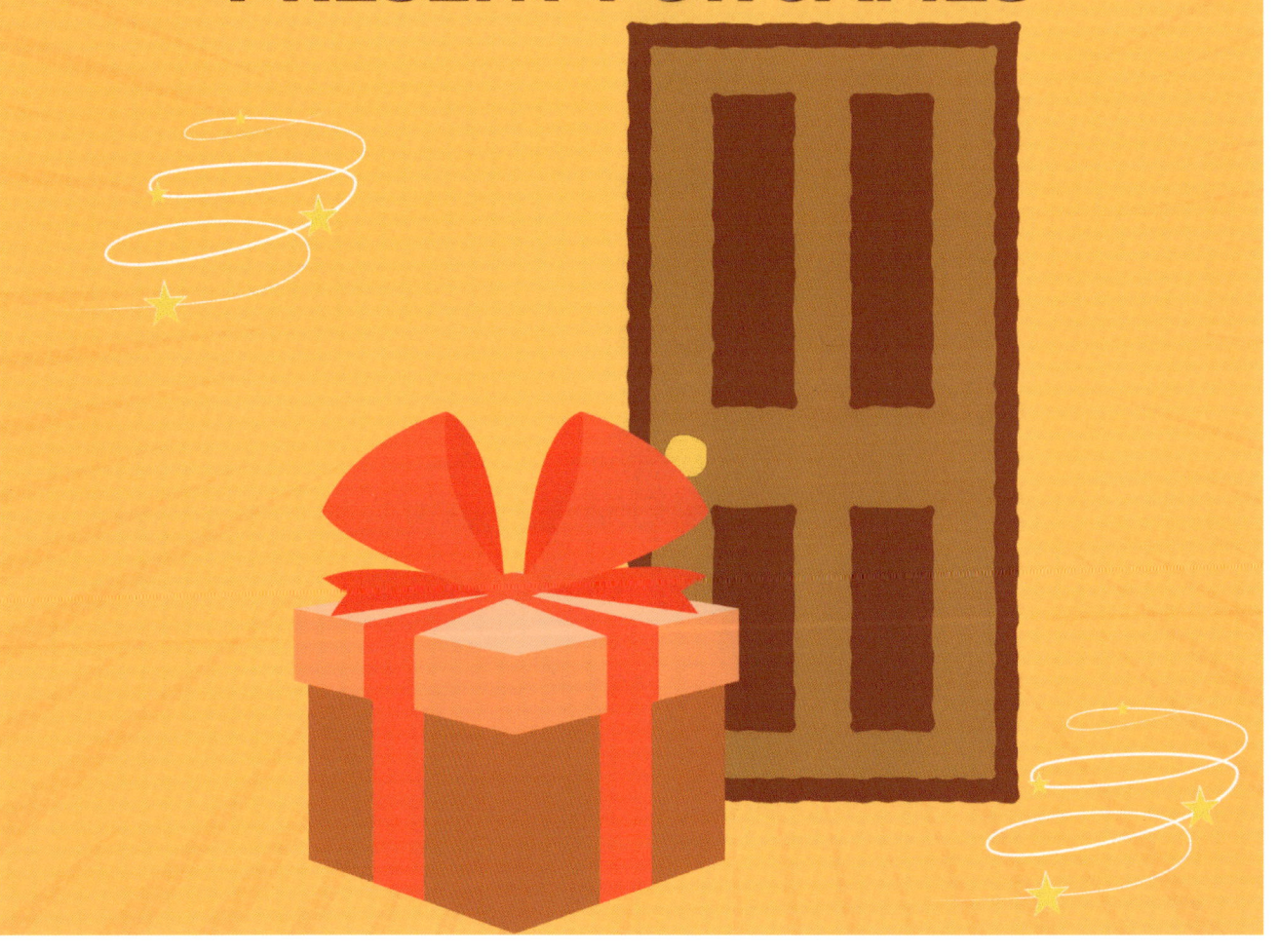

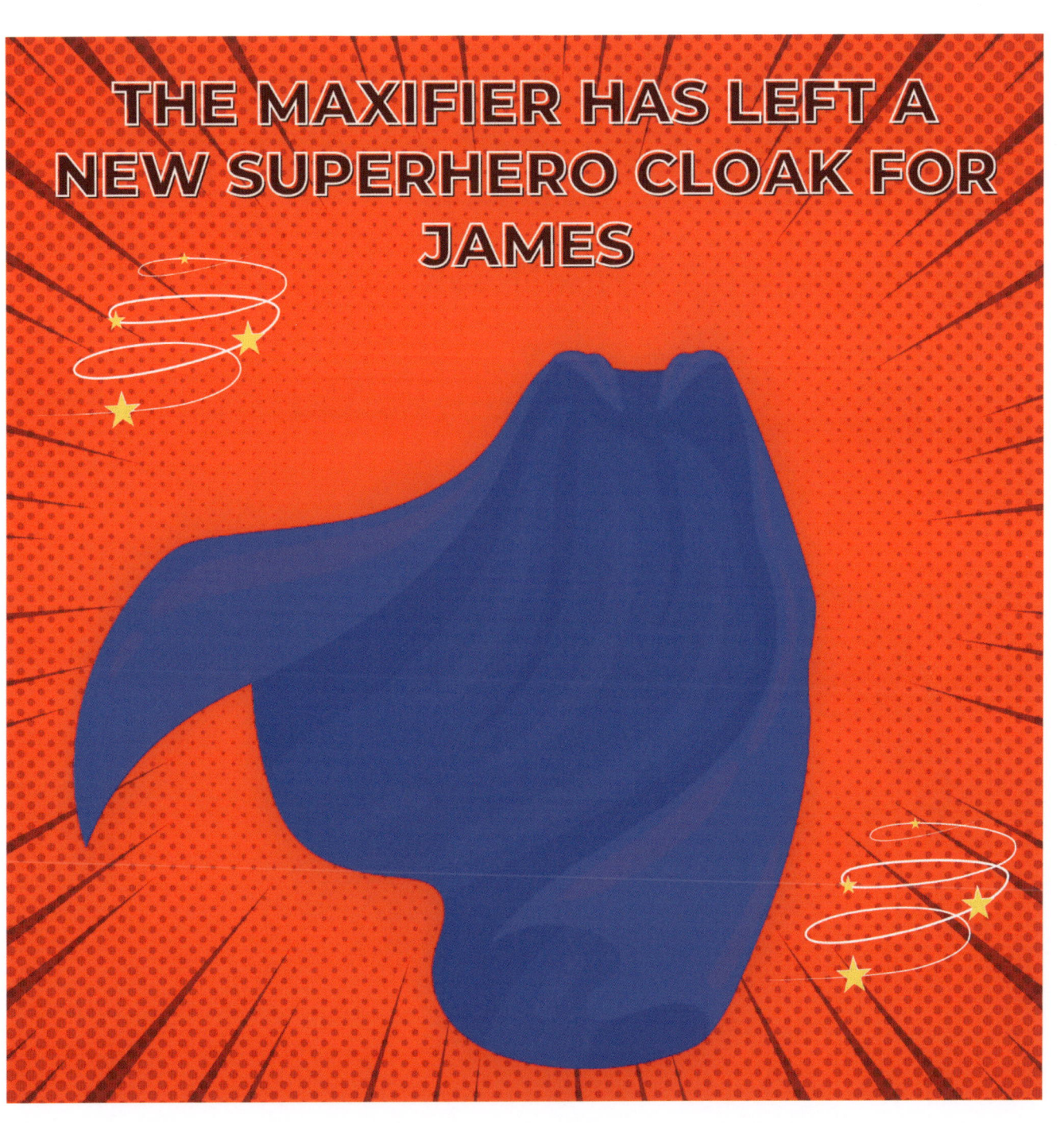

JAMES IS SO HAPPY HE WEARS BOTH CLOAKS

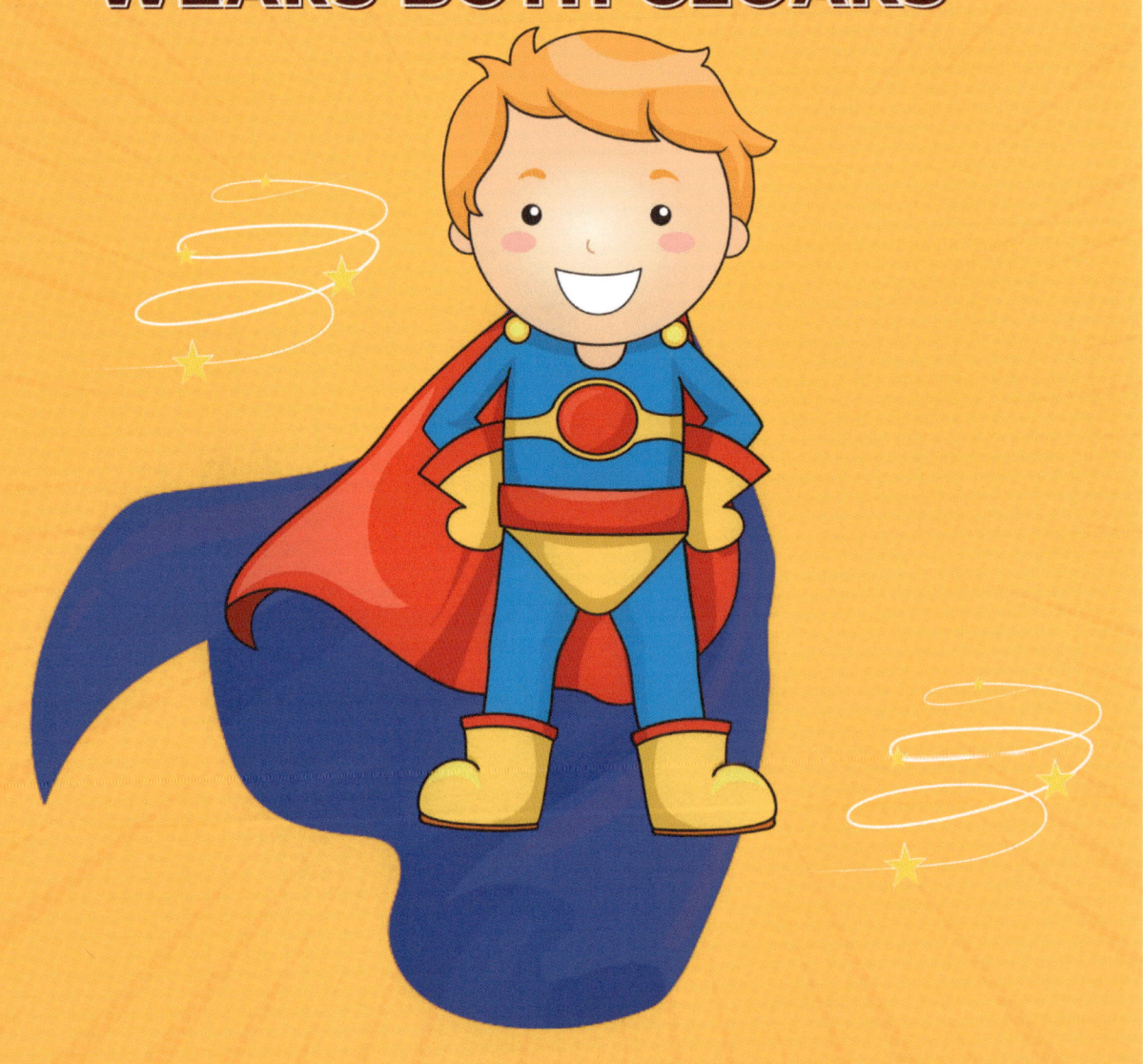

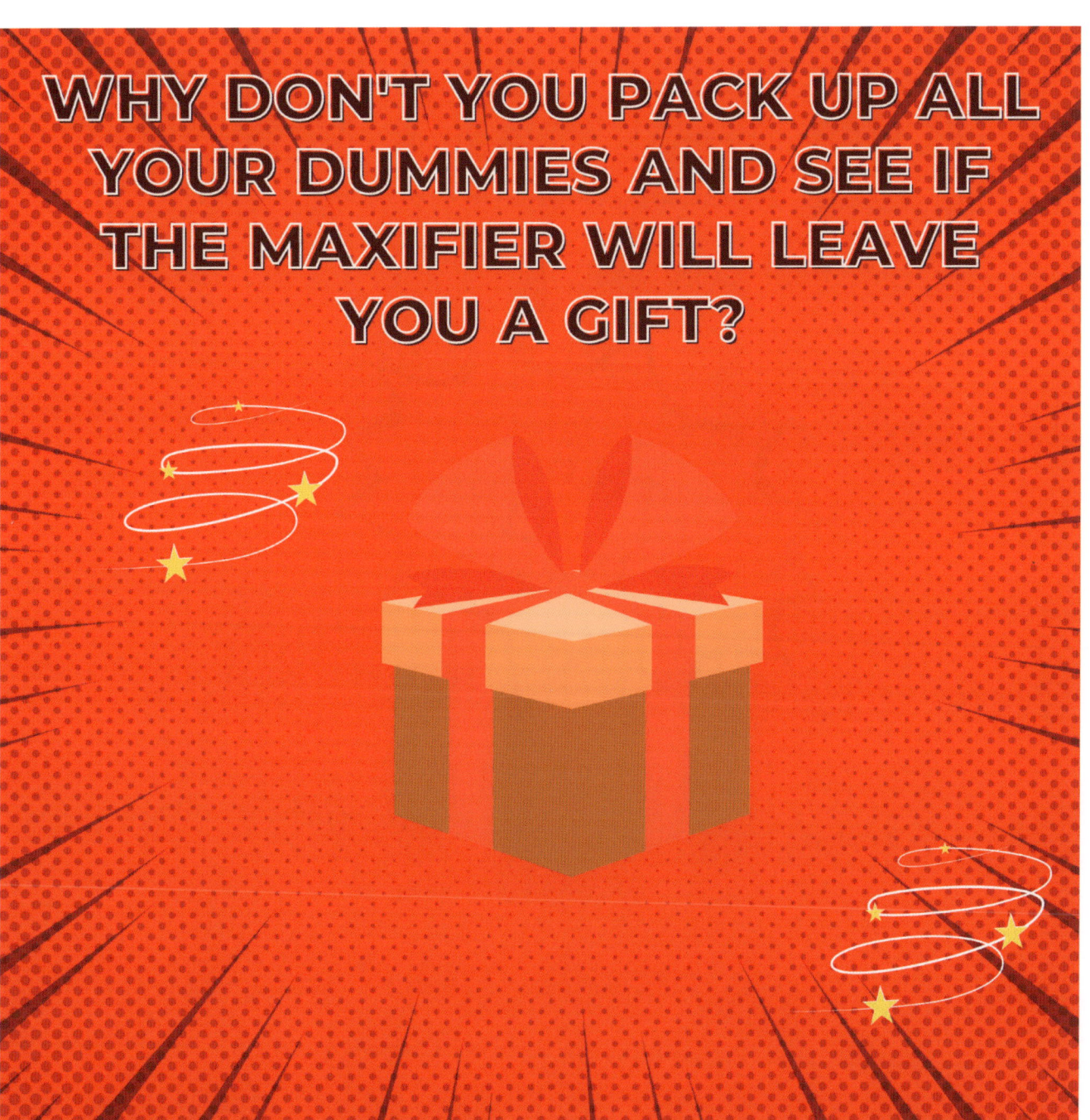

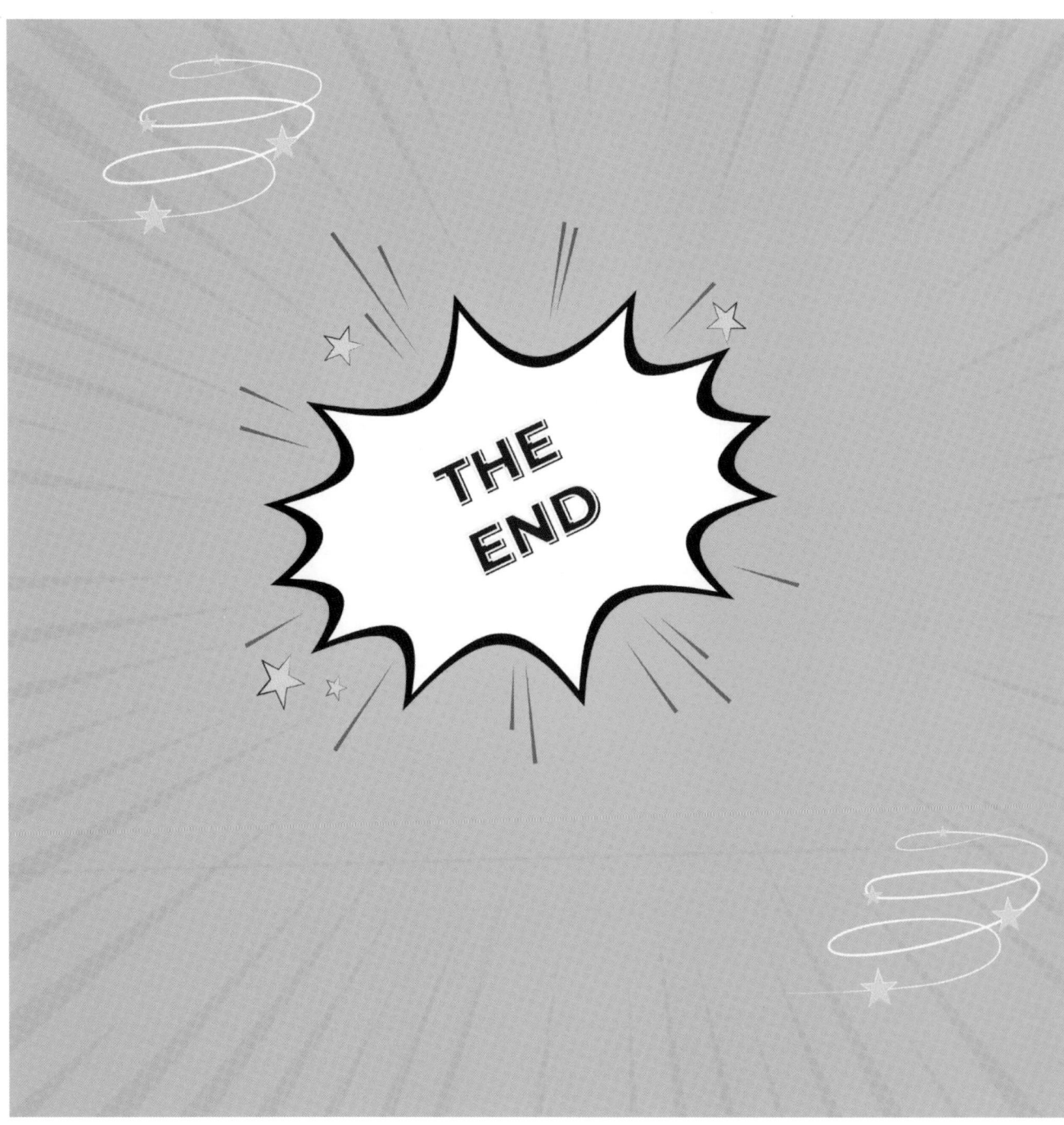

Printed in Dunstable, United Kingdom